COMPLETE WEIGHT LOSS

Step-by-step guide

to help you lose weight and remain healthy

Esther Ray

Table of contents.

INTRODUCTION

CHAPTER 1

Why am I putting on weight?

CHAPTER 2

Now, what do I do?

CHAPTER 3

Benefits of nutritious eating.

CHAPTER 4

The Benefits of Exercise.

CHAPTER 5

The practice of a healthy lifestyle.

CHAPTER 6

Top Dietary Supplements.

CONCLUSION.

INTRODUCTION

Will you ultimately say, "Enough Is Enough" at this point?

I'm prepared to embark on a path to a healthier version of myself; I won't offer any more justifications; and I'm going to effect change by losing some of those excess pounds.

Not!

If so, get ready to CHANGE YOUR LIFE AND QUIT THE FAT ACT!

The infomercials I see on Saturday morning and at night simply astound me. They advertise these tools and gimmicks that guarantee quick weight loss. How many of us have seen those "ab devices" where you rock back and forth while sitting and the fat magically melts away?

Have you read the screen's bottom-most, extremely small print? In essence, it informs you that for it to work, you must follow some kind of diet.

While following a very rigorous diet or another popular fad diet can result in significant weight loss, the main drawback is that these diets are not long-term maintainable.

In addition to the obvious harm to your health, I've come to understand that the phrase "diet" makes me think of limitations. One definition of diet, according to the dictionary, is "a routine of eating and drinking in moderation to reduce one's weight." Diets not working is not a surprise.

According to studies, the majority of overweight persons who start a crash diet quickly gain back the weight they lost.

Today, it is simple to fall prey to promises of quick weight loss made by some diet plans, "magic diet pills," and other "wonder weight loss regimens." But in all honesty, it is a bunch of nonsense.
Before you choose your course of action, there are a few fundamental truths you should be aware of.

First of all, be aware that there is NO magic cure for weight loss.
When this happens, their health is significantly worse than it was when they were initially overweight.

To be honest, losing weight hasn't altered much since humans first started walking on two legs. What has changed is how weight loss tips are marketed. You must ultimately have a negative energy balance.

How do you attain a balance of negative energy? You can first cut back on how much food you consume daily. The second option is to step up the difficulty of your workouts. Finally, you can combine the first two strategies. I'm done now.
Having said that, this book's focus is on tried-and-true food and exercise guide be guides there is no such thing as a miracle.

CHAPTER 1

<u>**WHY AM I PUTTING ON WEIGHT?**</u>

It sure is challenging to maintain an active lifestyle and consume a healthy, balanced diet given the pace of our modern lives, the advent of technology, and the comfortability of fast food. But even with a busy lifestyle, it can be done if you know how to do it.

We will examine the following in this book's first chapter:

1. The primary causes of weight gain
2. The people we must consult with once we have decided to lose the weight
3. How sticking to a schedule will help you lose weight
4. Weight-loss tips
5. As well as a host of other topics that will teach you how to finally lose weight and keep it off permanently.

The main causes of weight gain are excessive calorie intake and fat storage because we consume more calories than our bodies require each day. We all understand this, so why are 63% of Americans overweight or obese? The portions we consume today are tremendous, as you can see.

We are in a positive energy balance when we eat more than we burn. Essentially, we store the extra as fat. If we were still living in the caves and knew that we wouldn't have food for seven days, this could be a wonderful thing.

However, this isn't the case for those of us who live in western civilization.

• **You Aren't Sleeping Enough**. It may be time to take care of any sleep problems you may have if you are dieting and exercising but are still not losing weight. In the Canadian Medical Association Journal, two Canadian obesity experts note that there is growing data pointing to a connection between sleep and weight loss. The study discovered that those who stay up later eat 400–500 more calories!

•**Your metabolic rate is one**. After the age of 25, we begin to lose 10% of our metabolic rate every ten years. If you follow the instructions in this book for kettlebell training, you can stop this from happening. In other words, when we have more lean muscle, our metabolic rate rises because our bodies need to build more muscle to repair the muscle from the activity. We gain weight when we are sedentary because this doesn't happen.

• **Your eating habits are subpar**. People in the West are now 30 pounds heavier than they were 100 years ago, according to my research for this book. They consumed more fat, which is even more intriguing! They avoided eating manufactured meals. "If man-made, don't consume it," stated Jack Lallana, which sums it up perfectly.

You see, foods high in sugars, carbohydrates, and almost everything made with flour are making us an obese civilization. Fast Food Facts reports that the fast food business alone spent 4.2 billion dollars on advertising in 2009! We are overweight for a reason. A meal planner has been considered by many people to help point them in the proper direction.

• **Greater serving sizes**. This is common knowledge. I'll use quick-service restaurants as an example. Since I was a child, the size of soft drinks and fries has increased. Simply said, most individuals eat too much. This meal planner can help you understand what a portion should look like, as was previously said.

• **Physical activity, or lack thereof**. Western society is being destroyed by this. Today's children are the first generation to have a shorter life expectancy than their parents, according to designedtomove.org. The human body is built for movement. To reach and maintain a healthy weight, regular exercise is crucial. What you eat, how you eat, and how much you eat are also important factors. I'd like you to join Sergeant Slim as he trains to become the world's fittest man.

Control your intake. Use your hand to measure instead of weighing or measuring as a basic rule of thumb in this situation.

Men need two pieces of protein, whereas women only need one. Your palm would fit inside of a section.
Both men and women should choose a portion of carbs that is the size of their fists. Finally, fats that are about the size of your thumb include mixed nuts, walnuts, etc.

Protein that is the same size as your hand should be consumed by guys. The majority of people frequently underestimate how much they are eating due to this aspect. Generally, you should only consume a portion of food the size of your fist at a time because it is also the size of your stomach.

When you are 80% full, stop eating. This is a method that I use 90% of the time, and it will undoubtedly help you eat less. Consider portion management in this situation; there is no better method to manage what you put in your mouth than by eating less at each meal. If you do this for a year, you will lose a lot of weight.

Try eating more slowly and avoid eating while driving, standing, or moving. You should only consume food at a table. You should eat slowly since your brain receives a signal when you are full.
When you eat quickly, your brain does not get the signal, leading you to overeat since you do not feel "full." I know you're busy, but if you substitute a nutritious meal for one when you're busy, you could still be able to maintain a healthy weight.

Of course, monitoring your intake of fatty and sugary foods is another important step. To be balanced, we all need nutrients, including good fats, but consuming a lot of junk food and sugary beverages will significantly contribute to our weight increase. Processed foods are typically low in nutrients if they contain any at all, and high in harmful fats, salt, and sugar.

People frequently blame their hectic schedules for their weight gain. To prevent falling into any traps that would force you to make poor nutrition decisions, you must truly plan in this situation. Tupperware is a crucial piece of equipment when working out, as a well-known bodybuilder once said. I completely concur.
You can plan your meals for the week and get a shopping list for all the ingredients you'll need with a meal planner like the one in the link. Then, on Sunday, cook those meals using Tupperware, freeze them, and then remove one each morning. You already know what you will be eating for the day, so there is no need to think.

Breakfast can be challenging to fit in, so to avoid making a bad decision or going without food altogether, I suggest using a meal substitute.
Must I start a diet?

The quick response is "absolutely not" They are not long-term solutions. It's difficult to avoid falling for the excitement when the newest "diet fad" is heavily marketed, as we've already covered. This is precisely the topic covered by Corey Lewis in Sergeant Slim's Weapons of Mass Reduction. Think about a lifestyle shift instead of a diet because this will create long-term healthy eating and activity habits as opposed to a quick-fix diet.

Do you enjoy skipping entire food groups like carbohydrates or chugging down weight-loss drinks that just don't taste very good or fill you up?

Most people seem to begin a diet around significant life events, such as marriage, high school or family reunions, or the big one—New Year's resolutions.

If reaching a healthy weight is your main objective, I would advise you to complete your research and take into account Sergeant Slim's Weapons of Mass Reduction, which takes a more pragmatic approach. At least you will be aware of how to keep the weight off in the long run once you have reached your short-term objective.

Think SMART when setting goals.
You must have a cause for making any kind of adjustment to your regular daily activities before you start. These would be regarded as objectives.

Goals are crucial because, without them, you'll give up when things become tough. Perhaps you recently moved from a size 40 to a size 42 in pants, and you're sick of being big. Maybe your doctor warned you that if you don't lose 50 pounds, a heart attack is a serious possibility.
Your objectives must be sincere. Writing them down allows you to exhibit them somewhere and be reminded of them daily. The abbreviation **S.M.A.R.T.** is the formula I prefer to use.

SPECIFIC: Starting with merely a vague concept of where you're going will guarantee failure. You wouldn't merely drive to get to a particular location in New York City if you were planning to travel there, would you?
On the other hand, you would receive exact instructions before leaving to make sure you arrived at your intended location. The same goes for statements such, as "I wish to get in better condition," which are too general to be taken seriously.

It has no force behind it, and you won't even be able to tell if you've succeeded. How so? Technically, you would be in better shape now than when you started if you just lost one pound!

Get specific and determine what you want because it is obvious that this is probably not what you had in mind. Consider setting a goal like, "By the end of this year, I want to drop 35 pounds and fit into the same clothes I wore in college." See the distinction? If you use specifics like these, you will now be able to determine when you arrive at your destination.

MEASURABLE: Your aim needs to be quantifiable, which goes hand in hand with keeping your statement specific. Why does this matter?

Make sure your statement provides a clear response to the inquiry "how much" The solution, using the same example as earlier, would be 35 pounds.

To keep you on track, you can go even further with this. Create little milestones that you would like to reach along the route rather than just listing your main objective.
You might state, "I want to lose 35 pounds, which means I need to lose at least 3 pounds each month for a year."
This gives you a fantastic tool to monitor your development, which will keep you inspired. After all, a journey of a thousand miles begins with a single step, according to an ancient Chinese saying. In a similar vein, it's impossible to lose 35 pounds all at once, but you can do it this week!

ATTAINABLE:is self-explanatory, and you must keep your objective within the bounds of rationality. Expecting to run on the treadmill once and lose 20 pounds in a day is unrealistic. Instead, you need to divide your objective into manageable chunks that are aggressive enough to keep you working hard but still feasible.

If not, you might give up after a few weeks of falling short of your goals. It might be wiser to start with a lesser objective and increase it as you regularly surpass it each week.

REALISTIC: By definition, an attainable aim is realistic, yet there is a small distinction between the two. You might be able to achieve a particular standard, but you might not.

For instance, while reducing your body fat to 7 percent may be theoretically physiologically feasible, it might not be practical. Your objective should be to get in reasonable shape if you are starting as a couch potato or 100 pounds overweight. Trying to improve your fitness from where you are now to that of a triathlon isn't practical, and you risk setting yourself up for disappointment in the future.

The mere fact that something is feasible (achievable) does not guarantee that you will succeed (realistic). Therefore, try to keep your objective in the middle, and everything should work out for you!

I want to reduce my body fat percentage from 22 to 14 percent over seven months. However, keep in mind that a difficult activity could be made simpler because it will keep you motivated. Setting the bar too low may cause you to become disinterested. Only you can decide where the ideal balance lies, and if you feel like you need a little extra motivation in the middle, you can always raise your goals!

TIME DETERMINED:You have probably noticed that each example includes a particular period. This is crucial since without it, you won't be able to make on-the-go plans.

You would only need to lose 2 pounds a month if you gave yourself two years to reduce 50 pounds. You will need to quadruple that amount, though, if your goal is to lose weight in only one year.
Therefore, a crucial component of your goal is your deadline, which needs to be very detailed. Next, what?

Now that you have a specific objective in mind that you have worked hard to make compelling, congratulations! What's the next move, and how can you make the most of this? You need to constantly remind yourself of this aim by posting it somewhere you will see it every day, as was already indicated.

This will serve as a reminder of your goals and may also aid in the formation of new routines. It only takes 21 days to establish a new routine or habit, so after three weeks of healthy diet and exercise, life will be a lot simpler.

However, if you've battled your weight for a long time, your eating habits and sedentary lifestyle may be deeply ingrained in you. To break out of this rut, you might need to be assertive and attempt something a little insane!

Is a negative medical report what eventually motivates you to lose weight? Then display your medical records, test results, or even just a reminder of your poor state of health next to your written goal.

Why on earth would you engage in such a horrible activity? You see, if you're like most people, you'll want to quickly forget about this worrying development. This is just normal because you don't want to think about uncomfortable things all the time.

But you must do so because it might inspire you like nothing else in your life. It will become clearer to you that you cannot afford to waste this time when you see the test results or your doctor's note every morning.

Alternatively, you can have a more uplifting purpose, such as fitting into a reduced dress size for a forthcoming occasion. Why not provide an image of the contested clothing, or even the dress itself?

It may sound a little out of the ordinary, but seeing your objective there in front of you every day will make it simpler for you to say no to the donuts at work.
The image of that dress will be still in your thoughts when you're tempted to abandon your diet or skip your workout. Although it may seem straightforward, this works! Why not give it a try as you might start getting results that you have never seen before?

Get Assistance

You might believe that you have reached your conclusion at this stage since you have created a **SMART** objective and posted it where you will see it every day. Although this is a fantastic beginning, you still need one more thing to be successful!

You see, the reason why most individuals fail is that they don't set up a support structure to get them through the most difficult moments. These will unavoidably arise, and somewhere along your weight loss journey, you will feel like giving up.

You might simply be going through a difficult day at work, feeling sore from your most recent workout, or feeling unhappy to the point that you want to eat an entire chocolate cake! Whatever the situation, there will be a point when you require support to get you through a difficult period.

Who should you contact to form your support group? It should go without saying that you need a supportive partner in your weight loss endeavors. Since they probably see you every day, it would be excellent if you could enlist the aid of your spouse.

Additionally, you probably share at least one meal each day with them, allowing them to observe your eating habits as well. Unfortunately, your partner might not be open to change and might be hostile to your weight-loss strategy. They might also be unhealthy, but they aren't willing to change, therefore they will only be a bad influence. If so, you will need additional help from other friends or family members to make up for the support you aren't getting at home.

It is ideal to ask a friend who is already physically fit for assistance because they are aware of what it takes to keep the weight off. Additionally, they won't be enticed to skip workouts or consume bad foods, so they won't give in if you beg them to.

If you don't know someone like this, look for a friend with whom you can get in shape so that you may work together to shed the pounds. This can serve as a strong motivator since if you have a meeting at the gym, you can't miss your workout.

You will have additional motivation to maintain your diet since you will be required to tell them what you have been eating.

Get a Free Personal Trainer:This is similar to having a personal trainer, but without having to spend any money. Additionally, keep in mind that you may get in touch with me if you have any issues; I'm here to make sure you are successful in reducing weight.

Combining it All: You now understand how to create a fantastic objective that will keep you highly motivated. Keep your goals specific, measurable, reachable, realistic, and time-bound!

You will be able to accurately navigate and determine when you have arrived at your destination if all of these conditions are met. Then, just glance at it once a day or more to keep your new objective fresh. The next stage is to ask the assistance of your partner or a close friend to help you stay on the course anytime you are tempted to stray. You will be in a good position to achieve your weight loss goals if all of these factors come into play.

HOW DIETS FUNCTION

Simply consume fewer calories each day than your body needs to function to lose weight. We eat since our bodies must function. We will put on weight if we eat more than we need. Consider this: an increase in daily caloric intake of just 300 calories could result in a 20-pound weight gain over a year! We are consuming more calories than we need, thus this would be a positive energy balance.

In essence, a diet is meant to assist you in burning off those extra calories. Going ahead, consider a diet as a feeding strategy in which you would regulate your calorie intake. One strategy you might use to lose weight is to eat fewer calories. Don't let the fact that fruits and veggies are healthful fools you into believing you can munch on them all day. The opposite is true, as you can see. Keep in mind that overall calorie intake is what counts. Still, these meals include calories. You can choose the things you wish to consume and calculate how many calories you need based on your weight loss goals using my meal planner.

Many people think they won't be hungry because they have lowered the number of calories on their feeding plan. This might happen. Nonetheless, the hunger feelings can be reduced if you can eat every 2-4 hours. Divide the number of hours you are awake by three to get a quick formula. If you spend 15 hours a day awake, 5 meals should be your target. Using my meal planner, it was determined that you required 1500 calories total, or an average of 300 calories per meal, for the day. Your chances of success increase thanks to this meal planning.

A meal replacement might help you stay on track if your workload causes you to miss meals. Due to unforeseen circumstances, I do use these several times a week.

I do not recommend skipping any meals during the initial stages of your nutritional plan as this could result in what I refer to as "compensating." In essence, you will subconsciously tend to overeat at your next meal since you skipped a meal. This will inevitably result in eating more and putting on weight.

Diets generally fail because they are excessively restrictive for most individuals. Don't imagine that all you need to do is consume water and eat vegetables all day. Unfortunately, that won't work over the long haul. With my meal planner, you calculate your calorie intake and then create a weekly menu based on the foods you enjoy eating, not what some diet expert says you must consume.

A meal planner helps many people by eliminating the guesswork involved in determining the precise foods they should eat to lose weight. What can I eat? is the most frequent query I receive in regardregardingoss. It is now possible to respond to this query. a generalization

Discipline is one of the most crucial elements in maintaining a diet plan. It can take months or even years to lose weight through a balanced diet and get to your ideal weight. Yo-yo dieting can come from any extreme diet that encourages quick results. Yo-yo dieting is the practice of losing weight while adhering to a diet, only to subsequently overeat and gain back the weight lost.
This occurs because the diet he followed was excessively restrictive, banning many food groups and severely restricting his food intake.

He can't stick to this diet, so he gives in and eats more. Perhaps it can be the result of a lack of discipline once the desired weight has been reached. This is typically what happens when you follow an extremely high-calorie diet.

To prevent that, you should adopt a healthy lifestyle and learn to eat well, exercise frequently, and get enough sleep. It will be challenging at first to break bad behaviors. But if you follow your new eating strategy for at least 21 to 30 days, it ought to create a solid groundwork for success.

Your significant other will need to support you as you switch from an unhealthy diet to a healthy one. I've seen it happen far too often where the person who is closest to you will undermine your efforts. Why not convince them to accept your new feeding strategy? Making this modification will have a positive impact on their health even if they don't need to lose weight. The fact that my meal planner offers countless possible combinations is the final reason why using one is essential for success. How do I expect you to live on chicken and broccoli every day when I know I couldn't? You won't be bored because of the range of dishes available, including your favorites, and your chances for

Just keep in mind that you can get back on track the following day if you fall off the wagon and consume one or more meals that exceed your daily calorie limit. In the end, all that is required of you is compliance 90% of the time. You can't do this every day, but doing it once a week won't significantly hinder your efforts to lose weight.

Trade Secrets
The weight loss business is keeping several facts from you because they don't want you to know them. They are marketing fads, devices, and medicines to people who are anxious to lose weight, and their business is thriving as a result.
Regrettably, the only thing in most cases that is growing lighter is people's purses.

Few people who subscribe to one of these ideas succeed in losing weight and keeping it off, as many of these things do not work.

Some of These Business Secrets Involve:

Buyers are duped by the majority of advertisements for weight loss products. Most weight loss items that you hear about on the radio and see on infomercials don't even work as they are supposed to. Yet, with claims like "Lose the weight and keep it off," "Eat whatever you want," and "no diet or exercise required," people are persuaded to purchase these items. The general rule is that anything that seems too good to be true probably is

It doesn't necessarily mean anything works just because it's "scientifically proven" or "doctor-endorsed." Similar claims are also common, but they never disclose the location or authors of the studies so that you can independently assess their validity.
And anyhow, what does it mean? These "health professionals" frequently have a financial stake in the product, therefore they most likely skipped over the scientific research. Even if it was examined, they might not have adhered to reasonable review criteria. Why would you want to do anything like that and endanger your health?
A product's safety for consumers or ability to live up to its promises is not guaranteed just because the government permits it to be sold.
It's a common misperception that the government wouldn't approve the sale of a product if it would endanger you. Individuals often assume that the government must first pre-approve them, although this is frequently not the case.

There is no guarantee that products labeled "natural" or "herbal" are secure.
Also, some people believe that just because a product has natural components, it must be safe. Yet, businesses are permitted to promote their products up until the FDA obtains proof that they are hazardous.

It's important to remember that not everything you hear is accurate. You should avoid purchasing any items with exaggerated claims because many out there just do not live up to their promises.
Also, don't believe in the marketing of fad diets. It is quite challenging to maintain anything over time that calls for abrupt and drastic adjustments to your eating habits.

They will start you on a rapid weight-loss cycle, which is always followed by a rebound phase during which, in some cases, you may put on even more weight once your regular eating habits resume.

Also, it makes losing weight the next time you attempt that much more challenging. These diets offer no health advantages, and do you believe that there would be a demand for new ones if they all worked?
Also, you cannot rely on the money-back guarantee. You have roughly the same probability of getting your money back as you do of the product living up to its promises.

The ability to finally lose weight cannot be achieved with a quick fix or miraculous drug. You can almost certainly ensure that they won't work if the product makes such claims.

CHAPTER 2
NOW, WHAT DO I DO?

You must be dedicated to any diet to succeed at it. Only by adopting the proper mindset can you achieve success. Before you can go on to the next phase of your diet, you must first prepare yourself by understanding what stage you are in. It may not be seen, yet it is nonetheless present.

Pre-contemplation is the initial stage. You don't think of yourself as overweight. You don't feel like altering who you are. Only intense pressure will motivate you to look for assistance. Yet if that happened, you wouldn't give in; you'd just give up, feeling defeated by your situation.

Contemplation comes next. At this point, you start to recognize that you have a weight-related issue and brainstorm solutions. Yet you don't want to implement that remedy. You would simply consider it, knowing what steps to take to effect a change but never being prepared to do so. You won't get around to applying the remedy.

Preparation is third. You've decided to address your overweight issue once and for all. From dwelling on your issue to find a solution, you move on. You would also begin to envision a day in the future when you are healthier and fitter. But at this point, you're still not entirely committed. Considering that the remedy calls for a change in you, you would still have second thoughts about it.

Action is the fourth. You begin to take steps toward decreasing weight. You would begin making eating choices and engaging in daily exercise. It is the initial step toward accomplishing your specific objective.
Setting objectives is a must when trying to lose weight. Likely, your entire diet plan won't go as you had hoped if you don't set your goals.
"If you don't plan, you plan to fail," they say.

Describe the following:

A. How would you describe your present situation? Describe all of your eating practices, dietary preferences, and other factors that may have an impact on your ability to lose weight. exercising, etc.

B. Why are you trying to lose weight? This might be for a forthcoming occasion, the summer, or perhaps for a special someone. Write out the one, biggest reason that comes to mind.

C. What advantages do you gain from losing weight? As many as you can list. Health, more vitality, a partner's admiration, etc. are a few examples. This should be your primary driving force.

D. Your Purpose. Put this in bold to help it stick in your mind: "I want to lose XX pounds of weight in XX days." I think it's unrealistic to set a goal of more than 10 pounds every two weeks, especially if you're doing something similar for the first time. Be sensible. Writing "I wish" is required, not "I want"

Record everything on paper, then review it frequently. Placing it where you can see it will help. You will be continuously reminded of WHY you do this and what the rewards are once you start seeing it every day.

ONCE YOU TAKE ACTION, BE PERSISTENT BECAUSE IT WON'T BE EASY.

Exercising Your Comfort Zone

If you find yourself coming up with justifications rather than GETTING STARTED on an efficient diet, you should consider whether you want to lose weight. You must possess the ability to push past your comfort zone and, in the words of Nike's catchphrase, "JUST DO IT!"

Maintenance would be the last stage. You must maintain the momentum you had throughout the action stage. If at any point you stop being dedicated or supportive, you will revert to any of the earlier stages.
The final step of your diet plan is therefore the most crucial because you need to maintain your dedication over an extended length of time. There are various strategies you can employ to maintain your commitment.

Make a list of your initial motivations for doing this before anything else. To keep your focus on your goals, review the list every day. Avoid thinking anything unfavorable. Never and depriving are not appropriate words to use in your vocabulary.

You are just claiming that you only eat sweets "sometimes and in moderation" as opposed to "never." The word "starved" might therefore be changed to "choosing" when you decide to forego chocolate desserts.

Imagine in your imagination how slim you will be in the future, achieving all of your goals. Your commitment to the plan and desire to succeed will be further fueled by this visualization. Use this visualization every day when you get up and whenever you feel your commitment waning. Who Should You Speak With About Losing Weight?

Once you've decided to lose weight, you should involve a few other people in your weight-loss efforts. These folks may assist you in a variety of ways, such as assisting you in selecting a diet regimen, establishing objectives, and receiving motivation along the road.

A dietician: Because becoming a dietician is typically only possible after obtaining a medical license in most states and countries, a dietician will have a wide variety of information that can assist you in understanding your body and preparing a diet that will meet your specific needs.

Meal planners are a less expensive option for dieticians. My meal planner is a revolutionary new technology that has a patent pending. It assists you in building balanced meals using your favorite foods by working with you as if they were your dietician or nutritionist.

Most individuals have never learned how to exercise correctly, according to a personal trainer. This, in my opinion, is crucial if you've never engaged in any sort of weight training. I wouldn't sign a long-term contract with a trainer, and I'd want them to know my objectives and how they plan to support me in achieving them.

If you do decide to follow my programs, I would caution you to scale the exercises both for at least the first year, both in terms of weight and exercise duration.
Family and friends: I always dislike doing this, but I have a plan that I believe you can put to use quickly.
I detested telling folks whenever I embarked on one of my 100 diets. Because this was yet another diet I was starting, I thought they were judging me. Instead, say (if they ask) that you're just trying to eat a little healthier and that you're done with diets when you're at the dinner table during a party, holiday, or another special occasion.

This was effective for me psychologically for some reason. I think it will be successful for you as well.

Keeping Going Despite Failing

You will always fail when attempting to reduce weight or keep it off because you are only human. Those that are successful in losing weight did not give up when things got difficult; instead, they persevered and discovered a lesson.
"The tough get going when the going gets difficult"

The two main strategies for handling failure are those. Keep trying and picking things up.

Don't worry about the little things if you stray from your diet or skip an exercise day.
Don't allow it to stop you. Get it out of your head. Consider all of your good days rather than just one mistake. The healthier lifestyle choices you make, the more good days you have; before you realize it, the bad days are few and far between. Yet the key is to persevere and get through the difficult times. Consider it a cheat day, then move on. This is how you persevere; it's okay to fail for a day, but don't allow it to turn into a week, then a month.

To deal with failures, you must learn to accept them as a natural part of life.
The next step is to take lessons from your errors.

When you fail, view it as a teaching moment. Just like in business, when you try something and fail, you learn what doesn't work.

The same holds for losing weight. Perhaps you should abstain from drinking if you find that every time you drink, your new diet suffers. Reschedule your workout if you find that you consistently skip it on Fridays due to a late work meeting.
"I haven't blown it. I recently discovered 10,000 methods that won't work.
Theodore A. Edison

Together with death and taxes, failure is a given in life. Even if you could, you wouldn't want to since you can't prevent it. Your setbacks and triumphs both teach you valuable lessons about life. Don't be afraid of failing; just keep trying and keep learning.

Friend System
Adding some accountability to your routine is one of the best things you can do when trying to lose weight. How do you go about that?

Buddies System

A fantastic motivation is having a friend with whom to attempt weight loss. When you truly share your weight loss objectives with someone, you'll feel more responsible for achieving them.

They can also be useful because the person can understand your difficulties with weight loss. You can encourage one another by sharing both your victories and your setbacks.

A workout partner is helpful if you exercise frequently.

They can transform a dull jog or walk into a treatment session that also serves as an exercise. Bringing a companion along for a trip outdoors is usually more enjoyable!

Having a friend is also beneficial if you enjoy weightlifting. You guys may push each other while also encouraging and helping each other out with things like spots on heavy lifts.

Although it is terrible to say, you can certainly locate a weight loss buddy in your group in the modern world.

The simple conclusion is that working with a friend can offer encouragement, support, and the always crucial accountability you need to lose weight. Now go find your weight-loss partner!

Why It's Important to Have a Schedule
Setting up a daily training regimen is the following stage in organizing your weight reduction objectives. I find that 6 AM is a good time for me. It was challenging to wake up that early at first, but eventually, it became a habit. I'll list a few benefits of exercising at this time of day.

1) Your workout is finished for the day

2) You may spend the afternoon with your family, partner, friends, etc.

3) If you are delayed at work, no problem. Your workout is done.

But they are the reasons I train at this hour of the morning. Friends of mine have admitted to favoring the late afternoon and early evening. Once more, time doesn't important as much as the fact that you must do the task.

Keeping Yourself in Check: By recording everything in a notebook or other form of a recording device, such as a smartphone, you are more likely to keep to your goals when you have a precise timetable to follow. However, if you do skip a workout or have an extra snack, you can mark it and resolve to do better the following time.

Understanding What You Do Every Day: Having a written schedule of when you should exercise or eat your meals might help you stay organized. By doing so, you can plan your activities around your training hours rather than scheduling them around them and simply skipping sessions.
This is simple to accomplish, and once you start doing it, you'll find that you miss your workouts more frequently until you entirely lose track of your fitness goals.

Lose More Weight: By sticking to a timetable, you are more likely to complete your workouts on time and ultimately lose more weight (or very, very few in the long run).

You will find it much more difficult to maintain a consistent pace of weight reduction if you frequently switch between diets, skip workouts, or skip meals, which confuses your body's metabolism.

CHAPTER 3.
BENEFITS OF NUTRITIOUS EATING

You may have heard a lot of people claim that eating a healthy diet is essential for maintaining a healthy body, but you need to understand what healthy nutrition entails and why it is so crucial. Define nutrition first.

"Nutrition is the process of giving your body all the essential nutrients that will enable it to develop in a healthy and balanced manner."

This is the simplest description of nutrition, and it informs you that you must consume healthy foods that are rich in essential nutrients. Your body may become strong and healthy with a proper diet, yet it can also develop and mend on its own. While a bad diet can weaken your body, make you sick, and prevent you from fighting off some mild ailments, it can also make you sick.

Calories consumed and expended

Most people who desire to lose weight have experimented with a variety of diets, supplements, and/or strategies. Several different weight loss strategies may be purchased. They're all making outrageous claims.

The harsh reality is that there are no magic medicines, diets, or workout equipment that will make weight vanish overnight. It all boils down to eating properly, maintaining good health, and consuming fewer calories than you expend.

That is the origin of the proverb "calories in, calories out." Make sure you expend more calories (out) than you take in (in).

This is a naive way of thinking, and a healthy diet involves more than just counting calories. We'll examine that in later chapters, but for now, let's focus on establishing a calorie deficit. You'll need some basic information to track this. You must first determine how many calories you naturally burn each day. It all comes down to things like weight and age.

How to Determine How Many Calories You Burn Each Day

Calculating BMR yields the following results: 66.5 + (13.75 x weight in kg) + (5.003 x height in males (kg) in cm) - (6.755 x age in years)

Calculating a person's BMR is as follows: 66 + 6.23 times their weight in pounds + 12.7 times their height in pounds in inches (6.76 x age in years)

BMR = 655.1 + (9.563 x weight in kg) + (1.850 x women's (kg) height in cm) - (4.676 x age in years)

BMR is calculated as follows: 655 + 4.35 x weight in pounds + 4.7 x height in pounds for women (4.7 x age in years)

This equation will show you how many calories you burn each day just from breathing, heartbeat, etc. If you didn't move throughout y, you would burn these calories (basal metabolic rate).

Once you know that figure, you must begin keeping track of both your daily calorie intake and expenditure. Due to the volume of data to be tracked, this might be challenging.

Not that you should starve yourself or work out nonstop. It all comes down to being conscious of what you put into your body and what you expend. Although losing weight can be challenging, if you can control how many calories you consume and burn, you can succeed!

Healthy Eating
The fundamental weight reduction principle, calories in versus calories out, has already been discussed. It is a fundamental guideline since you still need to be cautious about where you are obtaining your calories from. It's probably not a good idea to have two corndogs every day to reduce your calorie intake.

Although there is no official definition for the phrase "eating clean," in general it means:

"Eating complete, nutritious foods and staying away from processed foods and refined sweets" While it may not always be practical to consume only "clean" foods, if you are getting the majority of your calories from clean sources, you are doing excellent.

As processed foods are avoided when eating cleanly, fast food and junk food are automatically cut out of your diet. The goal is to eat as leanly as possible, so don't worry if you do consume some processed food.

These are some general pointers for healthy eating:

Study label reading! Read the nutrient profiles and ingredient lists on everything you purchase. When possible, pick whole grains. Whole grain does not necessarily equate to whole wheat. Often consume fresh produce. They are excellent entire sources of healthy calories. Increase your home cooking, cut back on eating out, and avoid purchasing microwaveable meals. These meals, despite being marketed as "healthy," can be very high in sodium.

For cooking, choose lean meats. It's okay to eat meat because the protein will help you feel satisfied and build muscle. Excellent meat options include fish and chicken. Steer clear of processed meats like hot dogs and bologna.

Whole nuts that are unsalted or minimally salted can take the place of junk food. Great clean recipes can be found online.

Don't worry about slacking off; allow yourself the occasional cheat day.
It can be challenging to eat healthily while out, but more eateries are starting to offer this option.
If you're extremely hungry, you might need to add some protein to a salad, though!
As soon as you can, begin!

Eating healthfully is a fantastic strategy to ensure that you not only lose weight but also Your general health is good. You don't have to try to turn on a switch and make the change overnight, but it isn't always simple. Clean up your diet if you're serious about reducing weight and improving your health.
Your best friend is water.

According to research, you should drink at least 8 glasses of water each day, but how much you need will depend on your weight. Your weight would need to be divided by 2. Therefore, a man weighing 180 pounds would require 90 ounces of water per day.

So why is water recommended by experts and why is it thought to be so vital to living a healthy life?

First off, it aids in the removal of waste products, which prevents dehydration and maintains the kidneys' good health. Moreover, it helps to speed your metabolism, which aids in weight loss. But in addition to paying attention to what professionals advise, you should prioritize paying attention to your body. Naturally, you will drink water to rehydrate yourself when you are thirsty. Depending on the type of work you do, you should aim to develop the habit of routinely drinking water or, even better, keeping a water bottle on hand, especially on extremely hot days as the heat makes you sweat and causes your body to lose water, which you will need to replace.

Depending on the type of work you do, you should try to develop the habit of regularly drinking water or, even better, keeping a water bottle on hand. This is especially important on extremely hot days because the heat causes you to perspire and your body loses water, so you will need to rehydrate.
Water has a crucial role in our lives because of this. In addition to having no calories, it is also the best and healthiest way to quench your thirst. Eventually, you might think about replacing fruit drinks and sodas with water during all of your meals, which will help you consume fewer calories and make you feel much better because there won't be any added sugar in them.

CHAPTER 4.
THE BENEFITS OF EXERCISE

I'll explain what works best for melting fat, like butter, on a hot stove in this chapter. Exercising

First of all, the human body is built for movement.

Exercise has several advantages besides the obvious ones of keeping a healthy body weight.

1) Fights illness

2) Enhances your mood

3) provides you with more energy

4) promotes sounder sleep.

5) Better sex as well

Seven out of ten persons, or nearly four out of 10, are not physically active regularly, according to a recent survey. You run the danger of developing heart disease, diabetes, and stroke if you don't exercise. Over 300,000 individuals have died as a result of this.

You should speak with a doctor before beginning an exercise program. If you've been sitting on the couch and not working out for a while, this is crucial.

There are many diverse perspectives on fat loss in the world today. Running is typically the first workout activity people do. In any case, it increases your heart rate and is also aerobic.

What burns the most fat is aerobic exercise, right? You might be surprised to learn that running isn't that good at burning fat. That's because once your body has grown conditioned by the workout, you frequently reach a plateau (Peele, 2010).

In contrast, I've discovered a technique that guarantees you never plateau by steadily increasing the challenges with each session. Also, it burns fat up to 3,000% more effectively than your morning run!

Why HIIT Outperforms Running?

It is an original strategy and is known as HIIT or High-Intensity Interval Training. It will cut the length of your workouts and burn up to nine times more fat than running (Cossaboon). It means it is 36 times more effective overall when combined with the fact that it completes in a quarter of the time. How is this even conceivable?

First off, you burn more calories because of the intensity of the workout itself. Even if fewer of these are exclusive, You benefit because the total is higher from fat.

The most astounding aspect of **HIIT** training is, however, the second way it functions. Your metabolism is increased for up to 24 hours after your workout is over. That implies that while you're lounging on your couch at 11 p.m. the same night, you could be burning fat!

HIIT was a great fit for me because I value getting the most out of my money. Also, you just need to exercise three times each week to start seeing the effects; you don't even need to exercise every day.

How does it function?

The HIIT technique employs a two-pronged strategy to produce results quickly. Instead of exercising at the same intensity throughout your workout, you'll use two instead, and choose several intensities.

Running at a reasonable pace is a nice illustration of the first, which is a moderate level. The second involves short bursts of high intensity, like sprinting at your utmost speed.

You should train at a slower pace for up to 2.5 minutes, followed by a quick burst of high-intensity exercise lasting 10 to 30 seconds. Repeat this template once more while returning to the moderate level when 15 to 20 minutes have passed.

Your metabolism will be in overdrive at the conclusion, and it may remain that way for several hours or the rest of the day. This means that when you exercise and while your body is recovering afterward, you are both burning fats. Your findings will be expedited as a result, and Start removing the body fat straight now.

Maintain Your Focus

But if you don't maintain your heart rate up high enough during your fat reduction regimen, you won't experience any of these wonderful advantages.

What rate should you aim for to get the most out of **HIIT**? Your heart rate should be close to your safe limit during the few times when you are working as hard as you can.

How can you come to this conclusion? First, subtract your age from 220 to determine your maximal heart rate. Next, while you are at the high-intensity part of your HIIT activity, you should aim for 85% of this number (Baker, 2011).

To hit the beats per minute required to provide the desired impact, you'll need to work harder than you probably imagine. You haven't worked yourself hard enough if you can still talk while doing this or if you aren't gasping for air afterward.

Melt away the fat

You'll have a potent tool to aid you in your weight loss program when you employ HIIT in conjunction with your target heart rate. Including this kind of workout in your fat reduction program will hasten your progress and improve your outcomes!

As **HIIT** enables you to go even further than traditional cardio training, it is a more effective strategy for burning fat. You see, the brief periods of vigorous exercise are intended for every time you are close to your limit.

Since you can't sustain this level for the duration of a workout, your energy expenditure will inevitably drop.

For instance, you might be able to sprint at your top speed for ten to fifteen seconds, but not for the entire thirty-minute session. You have to slow down to a quick run to get through the workout, which has different consequences on your body.
Add Kettlebell Strength Training to Your Routine.

Strength training with kettlebells is a useful supplement to your HIIT exercises. Women avoid the weight room, whereas many males rush to the gym. You could believe that this kind of workout will make you look heavy and muscle-bound rather than give you the slender appearance you likely desire.

Yet, weight lifting with kettlebells is a highly effective method of losing weight when done correctly. You will preserve your flexibility while also developing lean muscle with the exercise I've included, giving you a beautiful athletic look.
In addition to being advantageous for other reasons, load-bearing exercise has been demonstrated to prevent osteoporosis (Rogers, 2012). While walking on its own is sufficient to provide this effect for your lower body, To achieve the same upper-body bone-building results, you must lift weights.

Moreover, resistance training can increase your metabolism for several hours following your workout, which will further your weight loss efforts. Women must utilize the weight room and the potent kettlebell to the fullest to achieve all of these benefits.

Why Use a Kettlebell for Exercise?

A good question. I didn't fully get it the first time I saw someone practice with one. Yet after being asked to take part in an exercise, I was able to appreciate exactly how useful these tiny tips could be for becoming in shape.

Unless you've been living in a cave in Afghanistan, you've probably heard that kettlebells are Russian in origin and that the fitness industry has welcomed them with open arms.

Let's talk about the many benefits of training with kettlebells:

1. Strengthens you
2. Physical stamina Burns Fat 3. Loss of weight
4. Develop lean muscle.
5. Reduces Fat
6. Mental fortitude
7. Develops a powerful core and slender abs
8. No gym subscription is necessary
9. Exercise outdoors or inside

Kettlebells Give You Life Prep.
Several of us have engaged in particular event training. Up until recently, the military mostly practiced pushups, sit-ups, and 2-mile runs. The result was a group of men and women who may have exhibited muscular endurance, but who would crumble if asked to move even a small amount of weight.

Forward to 2013, General Physical Preparedness (GPP) has now gained mainstream acceptance in addition to the military. The short answer to GPP is essential that you condition yourself to work.
Lifting weights and exercising successfully both require certain fundamental skills. You can build those with the aid of GPP. This is why the kettlebell is such a potent weapon in your arsenal of exercise equipment.

You can achieve the best physical condition of your life by simply practicing the kettlebell swing, squat, and Turkish get-up. You'll be stronger, leaner, and fitter than you ever imagined.
The human body is only as useful as its core if you think about it. You are weak if your core is weak. To be ready for anything life may throw at you, put away those ab gadgets, stop doing crunches, and start working with a kettlebell.

The Best Kettlebell to Use
When beginning any kettlebell exercise regimen, this is a crucial choice.
Women should start with an 18-pound kettlebell and males with a 35-pound bell. These weights should start you off on the right foot when working out, and they are fairly heavy when done with the right vigor.
The only kettlebells you should take into consideration are those that Pavel recommends.
You may see them here:

Security First

I've said it before, but you must speak with your doctor before beginning any physical fitness regimen. Despite the kettlebell's relative "lightness," using it incorrectly can nonetheless result in damage. It's also crucial to warm up properly before beginning any of the exercises in this book. Start slowly and get familiar with the fundamentals.

Footwear

When utilizing a kettlebell, it's crucial to keep your feet flat on the ground at all times. Wearing "running" shoes with a boosted heel is not advised. You can get hurt if you don't stand up correctly as a result of this. To save a few dollars, you can wear minimalist footwear or simply walk barefoot.

Getting better through practice

I applaud your desire to get started exercising and your determination to strive toward getting the body you deserve. So for the first week, the only thing I want you to do is to watch the videos that go along with it; after that, I want you to do the kettlebell swing.

Even though I still practice it, the swing is the most crucial action while I'm not aiming for perfection, I do want to execute the action with good form.
You can find my suggested kettlebell workout in the following chapter. This has all the necessary graphics and directions for finishing each day's workout.

Kettlebell Exercise Program

No matter if you've ever used a kettlebell or not, be sure to pick a weight that you can move without getting hurt. Kettlebells are an excellent tool for getting in shape, but they must be handled with care. You will see the effects of this training after eight weeks if you follow a healthy diet and get enough rest. Before beginning any workout regimen, be sure to acquire your doctor's consent.

The exercise is intended to be performed four days a week. Mon./Tues., Wednesday as a rest day, and finally Thursday/Friday are my suggestions. Life happens, of course. As close as you can, follow the plan.

Each workout's outline is provided below, followed by more thorough instructions.

Prior Plank

A place to Begin a Front Plank
On your hands and knees with your back flat, this is the starting position. Exercise your abdominal muscles. Elevate yourself into the push-up position by placing your weight on your forearms and toes. Avoid rotating the trunk or sagging or arching the spine. Keep your eyes forward and your head up. The objective is to maintain this posture for 60 seconds. If you are unable to hold for a minute, try again. Breathe normally while performing this exercise.

FLEXOR HIP STRETCH

1. Begin with the right leg raised, both arms overhead, and the left knee on the ground.

2. Keep the position for roughly 10 seconds.

3. Change sides, then hold for 10 seconds on the new side.

Notably, this warm-up activity encourages flexibility of the back, quadriceps, lats, and other key muscle groups as well as the core. You should stretch your body out like this before engaging in any physical activity.

PUSH-UP

I am aware that the majority of individuals believe they can do a push-up.

1. Lower your body until your upper arms are parallel to the ground while bending your elbows.
2. Extend your arms fully, locking out your elbows.

The trick is to lock out your arms and fully stretch in the up position. Second, make sure your arms are parallel to the ground when you are lying down. For the full impact of this dance, move slowly and deliberately instead of thinking quickly.

Variation: To perform push-ups correctly if you are unable to do so as shown, use a kneeling stance. This is a logical development.

SWINGING A KETTLEBELL

1. Squat down and raise the weight while keeping your back straight. Just keep it straight; don't confuse this with a vertical back. Avoid arching your back.

2. Squat down and straighten your shoulders.

3. Decide to sit back rather than stoop.

4. Make sure your body is in a straight line and that your hips and knees are extended at the top.

5. The bell should never rise above the parallel for the Russian-style swing shown here.

6. Ensure that you have flat feet by going barefoot or donning a minimalist shoe.

Practice with light weight at first until you can execute the movement properly.

Turkish etiquette
Movement:
1. Lift the kettlebell off the ground with both hands while crouching in a fetal position at the beginning and end of the movement.

2. The foot and hand should then be set. Keep in mind that the arm is upright and has a straight wrist on the kettlebell side. To get ready to stand up finally, bend the knee on the side of the kettlebell. Your core and lats are both active and prepared to work. You have your opposite leg straight and your arm 45 degrees away from the kettlebell.

3. Lock your elbow and maintain it in that position throughout the movement.

4. Throughout the movement, maintain your shoulder in a "packed" position at all times.

5. Focus on each position as you slowly and smoothly stand up.

6. This is not a fast-paced exercise.

Warning: This appears to be quite simple. Up until you reach each position, use a very little weight (5 pounds) or even a sneaker. We used the shoe in my Hardstyle Kettlebell Certification course. I strongly recommend the sneaker.

1. Straddle the bell with your feet slightly wider than shoulder width for the **DEADLIFT** movement.

2. Kneel and grasp the bell's handle with both hands while extending your arms between your legs.

3. Make sure your shoulders are over the bell and maintain a straight back.

4. With your hips and knees extended and your chest raised, lift the bell off the ground.

5. Squat with a vertical back and lower the bell while maintaining a taut back.

A word of caution: Avoid arching your back. Before adding weight, be sure you can perform an air squat correctly without any assistance.

SNATCH
Movement:

1. Start with the Russian swing.

2. Gently catch the bell without "banging" it against your wrist.

3. You can accomplish this by "punching" to the movement's peak.

4. Your arm should be level with your head when you lock out at the top.

5. To finish a swing, lower the bell to the ground, then repeat as necessary.

Precaution: Keep your back straight and use a weight that you can control properly.

Learning the Rack: When I first started using kettlebells five years ago, a trainer demonstrated this to me. I advise practicing so you can master the motion. With the Rack and the Clean, it will be helpful.

Movement:

1. Take one hand to pick up the bell.
2. Use your second hand to position the bell by using it.

3. You are now in the rack position, also known as where the clean ends.

4. Lower the bell by "sitting down" and moving your hips backward.

5. By repositioning your hips so they are further back and not pushing the bell forward, the bell is falling completely vertically.

Precaution: Keep your back straight and utilize a lesser weight until you get the hang of the action.

Step one of **THE RACK** is to stand above the kettlebells. Drawback between your legs while holding a deep breath.

2. Push your hips backward and slightly bend at the knees as the kettlebells return (breathe in), allowing them to pass between your legs. Maintain a straight back.

3. Open your hips and move the bell forward by using your glutes as a rubber band. Breathe out as you push through with your hips until you reach a triple extension. While performing the exercise, keep your elbow tucked and the bells should land between your arms and forearms.

4. Your bells are currently stacked.

Precaution: Make sure your back is straight and choose a weight that you are capable of securely lifting.

Squat with two kettlebells in front

Movement:

The bells should be stacked when you start.
Just over your collarbone, position the handles.
3. Place your feet slightly farther apart than shoulder width.

4. As you sit down, take a deep breath and maintain a straight back.

5. As you stand up, let out a long breath.

Precaution: Take care not to arch your back. Be sure to maintain a straight back. Choose a weight that you can move safely.

CLEAN\s
Movement:

1. Place your feet slightly wider than shoulder-width apart and straddle the bell.

2. Your torso should include your elbow.

3. All of the work will be done by your hips.

4. Have the bell follow a straight path, which is the distance between two objects that is shortest.

5. Avoid bending your knees when taking the bell or "racking" it.

6. Try not to whack your wrist or forearm.
Straighten your back and pick a weight that you can safely lift.

PRESS\s
Movement:

1. Place your feet just wider than shoulder-width apart.

2. Clean the bell off the floor or remove it from the rack, then place it in front of your chest so that it rests against the outside of your arm.

3. Ring the bell while raising your arm straight up in the air.

4. Bring your chest closer to the front.

Precaution: Make sure the weight you're using will allow you to execute the motion correctly.

Movement: Waiters or overhead

1. Press the bell out to the side to start.

2. Ensure that your elbow and shoulder are "locked" in place.

3. Start moving.

Take precautions by making sure your path is clear and choosing your weight carefully.

Movement of a suitcase:

1. Deadlift the bell before carrying it, just like you would a suitcase.

2. Maintain level shoulders and a tight core without compensating from one side to the other.

3. To achieve the desired effect, a heavier weight might be needed.

Precautions: When taking up or putting down the weight, make sure your back is straight and not rounded. Choose a weight that you can move safely every time.

Rack Walk\sMovement:

1. The bells should be stacked when you start.
2. Make sure the handles are higher than your collarbones.
3. Position the bells close to your bicep.
4. Avoid letting the bells sag or droop.
5. Get moving.

Make sure your walking path is clear of obstructions and choose a weight that you can move around with securely.

Goblet Squat Exercise:

1. Take the bell by the horns, first.
2. Feet should be spaced at or slightly beyond shoulder width.
3. Lower yourself.
4. Maintain an upright posture with as straight a back as you can.
5. With the weight on your heels rather than your toes, your elbows should be inside your knees.
6. Take an erect stance.
Avoid rounding your back, and pick a weight that fits your capabilities.

Movement: single-arm deadlift

1. Deadlifts are performed, but with weights at your sides.
2. Bell should be parallel to your ankle.
3. Keep your back straight and bend at the knees and hips.
4. Stand up straight without adjusting for the unbalanced side.
5. Take a tall stance.

The back must be straight and unrounded as a precaution. To lift securely, choose a weight that corresponds to your capabilities.

The farmers' walk motion

performed using two bells at your sides instead of the traditional deadlift. Employ larger weights to make the movement difficult. Start walking for the allotted amount of time.

Avoid arching your back and choose a weight that you can transfer securely.

Swing from hand to hand in the following manner: 1. Start with a regular swing but release the bell at the top.
2. With your other hand, grab the bell.
3. Move with intention.
Take care not to grasp the bell if it is too far ahead; instead, let it go and restart. Choose a weight that you can move safely.

Snatching motion from hand to hand:

1. Snatch with a swing to start the movement.
2. Use the same hand to lower the bell again.
3. Swing the bell up again and take it in your other hand.
4. Reposition the bell and start the transition as necessary.
Be careful not to arch your back and pick a weight that you can transfer securely.

Month 1

Day 1

TGU-3 alternately on each side

KB walks overhead: KB deadlifts for 30 seconds on each side. 4x5 weight, pay attention to the hinge, and lockout Swing ladders: 4 sets of 8 repetitions each with 3 bells of various sizes.

Carry-on luggage: 3 sets of 30 heavier bells one-armed deadlift each arm, 4x5 4x8 swings on a single arm per side Plank 5x: 30

Explanation in Detail: TGU-3 each. Alternating sides. Here, you should concentrate on executing the motion at each point. Perform the left side first, followed by the right side, for a total of 6 TGU. Work with a weight that you can manage securely.

This is a deliberate movement rather than one that is executed quickly. For the first two weeks, using something as lightweight as your sneaker to learn the technique is perfectly acceptable.

O/H KB Walk each side for 30 seconds. Here, pick your weight wisely. For a total of 30 seconds, you will move with the weight overhead. Make sure you lock the arm that is above your head. Normally, stroll.
Deadlift using kettlebells 4 x 5. Choose a sensible weight, pay attention to the hinge, and lockout. You will perform 4 sets of 5 when it is written as 4 x 5. Here, there is no set amount of time for rest. Choosing a weight that is neither too light nor too heavy will Most likely, you'll only need to take a minute to rest.

Swing Ladders: 4 sets of 8 reps with 3 different-sized bells. Start slowly when using kettlebells if this is your first time. A 35# bell for men and a 25# bell for women is likely the maximum. Start with the lightest weight doand 8 twtwo-handedwings, then move to the middleweight and do 8 twotwo-handedings, and then move to the heaviest weight and do 8 two-handed swings. You will then rest and do it again 3 more times.

Suitcase Carry: three 30-second sets. I used my non-dominant hand first, followed by my dominant and non-dominant hands. Put the weight down, take a break, and then pick it back up if you need to.

one-armed deadlift 4 x 5 for every arm. Avoid using the arm not supporting the weight to compensate. Be sure to maintain a straight back. Do 5 reps with one arm, then 5 with the other. Repeat three more times after the necessary amount of rest. Choose a heavy weight to start.

4 x 8 single-arm swings on each side. Start with either arm, count to eight with one and eight with the other, take a break if necessary, and repeat three more times. Be sure the weight you choose can be moved securely.

Five times for 30 seconds each, plank. Most likely, you won't be able to maintain the plank position for 30 seconds. So, if you can only manage 10 seconds, then rest for 10.

Day 2

TGU: 2 seconds on each side, pause in each position for 5 seconds.

5x10 hip flexor stretches with two hands swings

one hand swing 6 goblet squats with 8L and 8R.
Perform the first-hand swing and goblets four times. Swings from hand to hand
20 swings, then enter 4 times in 30 planks. 4 sets of 30 to 45-second walks by farmers

Explanation in Detail: Turkish Get-Up Pause in ea. 5 seconds, 2 on each side.

Here, you'll take a moment to rest on your forearm, palm, knee, and while standing. On the way down, repeat the process. Concentrate on feeling each posture deeply. Make sure you choose a lightweight. For the first two weeks, it's okay to use anything as lightweight as your sneaker to learn.

10 swings using two hands. You will use a weight that you can manage safely and perform 10 repetitions. Do this four more times after a brief period of rest.

Stretch your hip flexors. Spend some real time stretching each side. Here, keep your complete body in mind.

8L and 8R swings with 1 hand, 6 goblet squats. Using the same weight, you'll perform 8 swings with your left hand, 8 with your right, and then 6 goblet squats. Repeat three more times after a brief break.

Do 20 hand-to-hand swings, followed by 30 seconds of planking. Before performing this movement for the first time, make sure you have practiced it. If you're doing this at home, There is nothing in the path that can be damaged. If the bell sways, let it go and ring it again. After completing 20 hand-to-hand swings, perform 30 seconds of planking before starting the next round of 20 swings. This will be repeated four times in total.

4 sets of 30 to 45-second FFarmer'sWalks. Choose a weight that is difficult but not so heavy that you have to set it down after 15 seconds. Set the weight down, take a break, and continue three more times when you reach between 30 and 45 seconds.

Day 3 TGU: Stand up, move around for 30 seconds, then return to your feet and continue moving.
4x5 KB swings at 30/30 for 10 minutes after a KB deadlift
Goblet squat for six repetitions, then at the bottom of the sixth rep, curl the kettlebell six times by the horns. Swing L, pause for 30, and then repeat eight times. Stretch your hip flexors

Explanation in Detail: Turkish Get-Up Standing Posture Repeat with the other arm after walking for 30 seconds. Do a Turkish stance, then stand, walk for 30 seconds, stop, and then switch arms. Choose a weight that is not too light but not so heavy that you cannot complete 4 sets to perform 5 repetitions. After completing 5 repetitions, take around a minute to recover before completing 3 more times. Make sure your back is Keep your back straight and inhale while going down and exhale while going up.

Swing the kettlebells 30/30 for 10 minutes. You will swing your arms back and forth for 30 seconds, take a 30-second break, and repeat for a total of 10 minutes.

At the bottom of the sixth goblet squat, curl the kettlebell six times by the horns. four times. You will therefore perform 6 goblet squats, sit in the squat, and then perform 6 bicep curls with the bell. 3 more times should be done. Don't use the weight here in a forceful manner. Choose a weight that you can curl rather than one that you can use for goblet squats.

Stretch your hip flexors. Here, pay close attention to a good full-body stretch. Accumulate 20 seconds on each side as best you can. This stretch is awesome!

Day 4

TGU, for a total of 10 minutes, alternate between each side.

10 swings with each hand
8R and 8L One arm moves.
Do ten goblet squats.
20 swings from hand to hand:
Walk 30 overhead L/R: Carry 30 suitcases L/R

The above should be repeated 4-6 times.

Full Justification:

Alt ea. Turkish Get-Up 10 minutes total of side. Be careful when choosing your weight because you will be getting up and moving from arm to arm repeatedly. Don't concentrate on speed. To carry out this movement properly, feel each step.

10 swings with two hands 8R & 8L Arm Swings: 1
Do ten goblet squats.
20 swings from hand to hand
30 seconds of overhead movement, L/R; 30 seconds of carrying a bag, L/R Four to six times each.
On this day, it is intended to perform exercises continuously without taking a break. After finishing a round, take some time to rest and refuel to finish 4–6 rounds.

Month 2

Day 1

TGU- if possible, utilize a heavier bell; 6 total, alternating 3 on each side.

1 swing, 1 snatch, then 15 seconds of overhead walking

During 15 seconds, 2 swings, 2 snatches into overhead walking.
3 swings, 3 catches, then 15 seconds of overhead walking
For 15 seconds, 4 swings, 4snatcheshes into an overhead stroll.

Goblet squats should be repeated five times, pausing at the bottom for five counts before rising.
5x5 Kb rack exercises

5 cycles of 30

Explanation in Detail: Turkish Get-Up Ideally, use a heavier bell. Performing six times, three on each side alternately. You should be able to lift greater weight now that you've been following the regimen for a month. Naturally, pick a weight that is safe for your level of fitness.

Swing once and nab it overhead while walking for 15 seconds.
15-second walk with 2 swings and 2 snatches overhead
15-second walk with 3 swings and 3 snatches overhead
Walk for 15 seconds while performing 4 swings and 4 grabs into the air. Repeat the previous step five times.

The exercise is performed as follows: You will swing, snatch, and walk for 15 seconds, repeat this motion four times, rest as necessary, then repeat the motion four more times. As little time as possible should be spent resting. Push yourself to the limit here.

Goblet squat, hold the bottom position for five seconds, and then stand up five times. You will perform a goblet squat here, sit for five seconds at the bottom, then stand up and repeat five times. Repeat this process four more times after taking any necessary breaks.
5 sets of 30-second kettlebell rack walk: Rack the weight, then 71 takes a 30-second stroll. Done four more times with a brief pause in between.

Day 2\sTGU 8 minutes total, alternate each side Clean and press 5x5

5x5 double kb front squats

Push-up four flawless form sets
30 rack walks, followed by 20 hand-to-hand swings. repeat four times. Full Justification: Turkish Get Up for a total of 8 minutes, switching sides. As a friendly reminder: throughout the Get-up, pay attention to movement rather than speed. Your core will work harder if you lift a weight that is a little bit heavier than you are comfortable with.

"Clean and Press" 5 x 5. Perform a clean, then press it. Repeat this for five repetitions, take a break, and repeat four more times. Compared to pressing, cleaning will be significantly more effective. Based on this motion, adjust the weight of your press.

5 x 5 Double Kettlebell Front Squats Make careful you rack the weight, maintain a straight back, perform 5 reps, then rest for 4 more. Choose your weight carefully.

Push-Ups Four sets of flawless form. This puts your mental fortitude to the test. Push-ups should be performed as many times as you can while maintaining perfect form. Keep track of how many push-ups you complete so you can see your progress over the following three weeks. Here, emphasize form over speed. Push yourself to the limit here.

30 seconds, 20 swings, 20 hand-to-hand swings Rack Walk four times. To do this, attempt to use a consistent weight. Do 20 swings with each hand, 20 swings from hand to hand, and then rack walk for 30 seconds, 3 additional times, taking breaks as necessary. Keep the break as brief as possible.

Day 3

4 times in 30 seconds, each arm, overhead walk 4x30 each arm, 4 suitcases

10 arm swings, one 10 snatches in L/R 20 hand-to-hand snatches, L/R

repeat four times.
2 hand swings totaling 8 minutes 40/20 Full Justification:
Four 30-second overhead walks with each arm Suitcase 4 times for 30 seconds on each arm.
10 Arm Swings: 1 10 snatches left, 20 hand-to-hand snatches right, repeat four times.

Without stopping, move from one exercise to the next. Before attempting this, you should be proficient at hand-to-hand snatches. After finishing a round, take a little break to collect your breath before performing it three more times. Push yourself to the limit here!

Then:

2 Hand Swings at 40/20, total time 8 minutes. Do two-handed swings for 40 seconds, then rest for 20 seconds before repeating the exercise eight times.

Day 4

1 TGU per arm.
20 a two-handed swing
10 R and 10L One arm moves.
Eight goblet squats
Snatches in 8L and 8R

2 TGU per arm. 30 rack walks

For a time, repeat 4-6 times.

Full Justification:

Turkish Get-Ups, one for each arm. Here, test your mettle!
20 Double-handed swings
10 Left and 10 Right 1 arm movement
Goblet squats: 8
8 Left and 8 Right Snatches
Turkey Get-Ups, two Every Arm Rack Moves a minute For a time, repeat 4-6 times.
Notes: The get-ups should not be completed quickly. Consider each position. With a difficult weight, switch exercises, take breaks, and aim for four to six sets.
You can always restart the training program at week 1 if you've already finished the first eight weeks. You can reduce your rest periods and add more weight. In the future, I'll design more challenging kettlebell exercises.

CHAPTER 5

THE PRACTICE OF A HEALTHY LIFESTYLE.

Knowing how to maintain your desired weight can help you avoid wasting all of your hard work once you've achieved it. When you reach the point where you have accomplished your weight loss target, the knowledge you have gained in advance will be helpful. You want to keep up your newly discovered healthy lifestyle and would not want to mar the celebration you will want to have.

Never skip a meal! Keep in mind that your metabolism will interpret this as a sign that you are starving and start to store fat as a reserve. Make sure you continue eating your meals as you have been planning them. Furthermore, skipping a meal at one point during the day may result in overeating later on when you are simply too hungry.

Continue to eat a variety of meals. This will make it easier for you to continue getting all the vitamins and nutrients your body needs to stay healthy. It will maintain your body healthy, give you energy, and safeguard your body doing so. Whole grains, fruits, vegetables, and lean proteins are among the options you have.

Keep up your workouts! Don't become complacent and stop working out right away. You now know what form of exercise is best for you and presumably how to do it.

If you were under a personal trainer's instruction, you should occasionally switch things up. It's a good idea to switch up your regimen occasionally to prevent boredom and keep your body on its toes. You will continue to stay in shape, feel strong and healthy, and you will further protect yourself from sicknesses when you combine your cardio and strength exercise with a good diet.

Your calorie consumption each day. Many people ponder whether they should immediately boost their daily caloric intake. It is usually best to go gently, though.
Start with just 250 extra calories per day. Check your weight once a week. Most likely, you still have some further weight to lose.

If so, consume an additional 250 calories, then weigh yourself a week later.

When you weigh yourself at the end of the week, keep going until you see that it hasn't changed. If you've gained a little, reduce your calorie intake by 100 at a time until your weight stabilizes and stays the same from week to week.

Continue to sip on the water! To keep your body functioning properly, remember to drink at least eight glasses of water daily. Water aids digestion and gives you mmaldigestionurally dnatnaturallyody. You will also maintain your health and hydration.

Continue to eat frequently. You have probably already figured out that eating five to six modest meals a day is a smart idea because it keeps your metabolism going and leaves you feeling satiated.

It is crucial to keep doing this as well since, if this was an issue in the past, you don't want to fall into the trap of raising your portion sizes once more. One day you'll find yourself right back where you started. You will at the very least put on a lot of the weight you worked so hard to lose again.
Keep the unhealthy food outside. Why destroy your new healthy routines by reverting to your old behaviors and overindulging in junk food?

You've learned how to satisfy all of your cravings with delicious, nutritious foods. Maintain a daily diet of fruits and vegetables of at least six to eight servings.
Take your vitamins each day. Do not stop taking your daily vitamin supplements. You can ensure that you get all the vitamins you need each day by doing this, which will also help you keep a healthy weight.

The Guidelines for Remaining Healthy
Nobody wants to assume they will contract a serious illness; everyone wants to enjoy long, healthy lives. There are measures to help safeguard ourselves that can help make our lives full and healthy overall, even while we can't forecast or prevent every incident.

The first thing you should think about is prevention and early detection. Most individuals hate getting their yearly physicals or even going to the dentist every six months for a cleaning. Yet, following these checkups and finding competent doctors will help you stay healthy because they can spot things that you can't.

Understanding your family history is essential because your doctor can monitor your symptoms and perform routine tests if there is a history of cancer or heart disease in your family.
Respect the company you keep. Spend time with the people who are always there for you, such as your husband, kids, extended family, friends, and coworkers.

Cherish your interactions with others and uphold wholesome friendships. You need these connections to feel fulfilled in life.
Sleep for eight hours. Even though many people find this one challenging given how busy our lives can become, it is crucial to living a happy and healthy existence.
Discover a skill you excel in. Everybody has moments when they should be doing something they enjoy, and most of the time, these moments call for their best abilities. Typically, this also gives us a positive inside feeling and may even be calming and stress-relieving.
Don't dismiss your tension; manage it instead! Everyone experiences some form of stress.

thus we must manage our stress so that it doesn't outgrow control and take over our lives.

You can become physically ill when you are plagued by anxiety and stress in several ways. Regular walks can help you relax and check that your calendar is not too full or that you are not allowing other people's schedules to control your day.
Achieve equilibrium in your life. Try not to let work overtake you or attempt not to take on too many projects. Establish a balance so that you can still take pleasure in all the other things in your life, such as your interests, friends, and family.

Even though times can be difficult financially, it is still crucial to make time for your family, whom you work so hard to protect and provide for.
The Benefits of Maintaining Health

The advantages of maintaining good health are endless. It's not only that you can fit into that new dress and are content with the way you appear. Your overall physical, mental, and social well-being are all impacted by your level of health.

Your Physical Health: Maintaining good physical health will benefit you in all respects. It not only enables you to participate in daily tasks like walking, moving, and bending, but it also makes it possible for you to physically care for those who depend on you in your immediate family.

Avoiding diseases that may have been prevented and would have been very expensive can be financially advantageous.

Your Mental Health: Your physical health will be impacted if your mental health is poor. A lot of people are unaware of how crucial their mental health is to their general well-being. You risk becoming ill if you let stress overwhelm you or take control of your life.

The chance of having a heart attack or stroke increases if you are under stress. You must find healthy strategies to manage your stress, such as through exercise, meditation, or counseling. Avoid handling stress in bad ways, such as by smoking, drinking, or eating unhealthful foods.

Disease Prevention: Maintaining overall health and remaining healthy requires eating a balanced diet. Your health may be directly affected by the foods you choose to eat.

Phytochemicals are crucial for your health and may help ward off conditions including high blood pressure, certain types of cancer, diabetes, and heart disease. Just specific foods, like berries, spinach, olives, and kale, contain them.

Have a low-fat diet rich in whole grains, fruits, and vegetables to assist safeguard your cardiovascular health.
Long Life: Maintaining a healthy lifestyle can play a significant role in your ability to live a long and active life. Even while you can't prevent all health issues and some of them are beyond your control, leading a healthy lifestyle can help you avoid many of the more serious ones.

Having a healthy lifestyle that includes managing your diet is crucial because chronic diseases like diabetes, heart disease, cancer, and stroke are the major causes of mortality.

Maintaining a healthy weight, how much you exercise, and how you handle stress in your life can all have a significant impact on preventing these diseases.

Maintaining a healthy lifestyle can also lift your spirits, increase your sense of worth, and sharpen your mind. You will be more physically fit, have more endurance, and be able to sleep better at night.

Improved digestion and decreased blood pressure are two additional advantages of leading a healthy lifestyle. Maintaining good health can also help you reduce or completely get rid of back discomfort and difficulties, as well as improve your balance and coordination, posture, and resting heart rate.

CHAPTER 6.
TOP DIETARY SUPPLEMENTS

Things to Check Out
Finding a firm you can rely on and one you can trust to deliver the quality you are paying for is crucial if you want to advance in the development of your physique or if you're interested in the greatest diet supplements and cutting-edge anti-aging supplementation.
We have all probably had the unpleasant experience of being pressured into purchasing useless supplements in vitamin stores. This is the reason I decided to join Prograde Nutrition.

It's a serious decision to buy supplements that might help you achieve your fitness objectives, and Prograde seems to take it very seriously as well.
What Motivated Prograde to Start Selling Supplements?

Prograde was founded in reaction to the unethical business methods that are so prevalent online and in vitamin stores in the real world. It appears like everyone wants our money at these brick-and-mortar vitamin stores and internet retailers, but they won't offer us the quality we are paying for.

The biggest issue with purchasing the "greatest diet supplements," as many pushy sellers refer to them, is that many of the substances aren't as pure as they could be.
This is a waste of your money and valuable time that could have been put to better use in achieving your objectives.

Excellent business ethics and thorough research.

Most of the products you buy from a supplement store are often backed by made-up research, which is nothing more than a covert sales copy meant to persuade you to buy their products.

After reading hundreds of product labels and their sales copy—this was meant to be "research"—I realized there had to be something different. Something better, with actual people engaged in assisting me in locating the top multivitamins, diet supplements, and other health-related products that might help me achieve the advantages I was seeking.

The thing that most impressed me about Prograde was the fact that, before they started, they employed a renowned nutritionist to assist in creating their product range.

In reality, they only permit certified fitness instructors and health specialists to endorse their goods.
This is extremely dissimilar from what we see online when products with phony evaluations steer you toward purchases that are just made to enrich the seller.

Going to a typical vitamin store has got to be the most annoying experience.

Added justification for using Prograde

With Prograde's "Zero Risk" policy, I am also allowed to test any of their products for a full 60 days without taking any risks. This company is a fantastic resource for high-quality multivitamins for both men and women, in my experience.

Unfortunately, the quality of our food sources is declining. We need to discover a reliable source that we can trust and that also stands by what they say to maintain optimal health and vitality, which is essential for enjoying life.

It has never been more crucial in history to take supplements to maintain good health. You will recall the moment you first heard the name "Prograde" if you care about your health as much as I do.

Why You Need Daily Vitamin Supplements

Everyone aspires to look their best. This is why taking vitamin supplements every day can be the answer. The fact is that you are undervaluing yourself if you simply rely on food from the grocery store to meet all of your daily nutritional needs.

Though many find it difficult to accept, this is the case.
Furthermore, daily vitamin supplements should be a part of your diet if you want to burn the fattest possible. This will give you the advantage and help you get there more quickly.
In this article, we will address both men and women in separate sections so that you, too, can be delivered from the synthetic vitamin supplements found in grocery stores every day that do nothing more than pass through your system with no benefits at all, much less giving you a competitive edge in fat loss.

Why You Need Vitamins every day, But Specifically For Women
In actuality, there aren't many naturally derived vitamin pills that are made for a woman.

Finding daily vitamin supplements that may meet the extremely special needs and desires of women has, up until now, been exceedingly difficult.

A vitamin that may support your hormone balance, boost mood, and increase energy is literally like a gem in the rough.

The necessity of providing your body with daily vitamins at every stage of your life is obvious if you're a woman who cares about both how you look and feel.
You could have some quite serious health issues as you age if you don't consume all of your daily recommended servings of fruits and veggies.

The need to restore calm and balance to your life through daily vitamin supplements is now a reality because stress has grown far too prevalent in our culture.
Because it is not synthetic like 99% of the vitamins you buy in both online and offline places, you can forget about experiencing nausea when taking this new breed of the vitamin.

Did you know that if you don't consume at least 10 servings of fruits and vegetables every day, your health would suffer? Because of how difficult it is to ensure that we eat enough food and acquire the nutrients we require daily given our schedules, supplementing has become very popular.

And finally, a vitamin made specifically for women ought to assist you in replacing the nutrients you lost during exercise and in burning fat so that you might lose weight. In addition, this vitamin ought to give you the essential nutrients you require each day, whether or not you exercise that day.

A top-notch dietician would be required to create such a vitamin. I am aware of the vitamin because I am a partner of Prograde Nutrition.

A benefit that is missing from nearly every multivitamin supplement you discover on the market today is daily vitamin supplements that can give you the essential components you need to boost your metabolism so you can burn fat more quickly and develop that six-pack faster.

When you're attempting to eat enough food throughout the day to provide your body with what it needs, getting the right fatty acids, vitamins, enzymes, and amino acids happens only once in a blue moon. For this reason, as a partner of Prograde Nutrition, I wanted to share this information with you.
liquid diets for weight loss

Why Not an Alternative Meal?

Since you are probably undereating, I wouldn't advocate liquid weight loss plans as a first option if you are having trouble shedding fat. eating insufficiently? Certainly, many people are perplexed by this since they believe that cutting calories will result in weight loss.
These are only partially accurate, though. During 10 to 14 days, eating less is effective while your body "figures out" what you're trying to achieve. Because of this, some people "cycle" their caloric intake every 7 to 14 days. But we'll talk about that at a later time.
After that, homeostasis takes over and your body slows down your metabolism, causing you to consume fewer calories.

This is sometimes referred to as the "yo-yo dieting syndrome" because of the weight gain that follows these kinds of diets.

If you keep doing this, your metabolism will become damaged, which will make it extremely harder for you to lose weight. Several people have tried pure liquid diets as part of their weight loss efforts, but I would not advise or support this.

Why? Is There a Solution?
Yes. I want to tell you about a fantastic meal replacement supplement that I use as a partner with Prograde Nutrition.
You see, maintaining a trim figure requires balance. Why not indulge in a nutritious meal replacement in between meals rather than a "liquid weight loss diet"? How come this is important?

Because increasing your metabolism is the key to reducing weight.
In a nutshell, this means consuming enough calories that your body has to work nonstop throughout the day to process the food you're feeding it. Furthermore, can you picture consuming only liquids for every single meal while on a plan to lose weight? Please offer me genuine food, unless your jaw is wired shut.
Your body can become a calorie-burning machine as a result.
Here's Where The Equilibrium Enters The Picture

You won't achieve your goals by simply eating at a fast food restaurant for six meals a day. Fast food has an excessive amount of saturated fat that will do more harm than good, as well as too many empty calories, which are calorie-rich but low in nutrients.

Eating 5 to 6 small, healthy meals per day will help you take advantage of the thermic effect of food, which simply refers to the fact that eating causes your body to work harder and raises your metabolic rate even when you are not eating. This will help you lose fat and keep it off.
Watch out because you might start losing some of that extra fat as your metabolic rate rises!
Most likely, a liquid diet for weight loss won't produce the same outcomes.

Which shake is a meal replacement?
Taste is crucial in the first place. Anyone's compliance will decrease if they have to consume anything unpleasant, regardless matter how much protein and vitamins it provides.

The thermic impact of food, which simply refers to the fact that eating makes your body work harder and increases your metabolic rate even when you are not eating, can be benefited from by eating five to six short, healthy meals per day. This will assist in your long-term fat loss.
Be careful because when your metabolic rate increases, you might start losing some of that extra fat! A liquid diet for weight loss probably won't result in the same results.

Which smoothie can you use to substitute a meal?
Taste is important first and foremost. No matter how much protein and vitamins are in something, if someone has to eat it, their compliance will suffer.

No. NO artificial sweeteners, please. Check.

I can't even begin to count how many times I have located the necessary materials only to discover this at the bottom. Phenylketonurics: Phenylalanine is present! This is aspartame, which has a variety of negative effects.

This is something I need to avoid if I plan to drink something two to three times per day. Artificial sweeteners' headaches are something I can live without. I need something natural if I'm doing this for my health.

Low Fat "I'm trying not to drink it, but to lose it!"
Recently, there has been a lot of meal replacement shakes with a lot of fat. Why? The manufacturers are aware that it improves the taste, yet What they fail to mention is that you will have to watch how much unhealthy fat you consume at other meals, which will throw off your daily requirements. This requires way too much calculation, and I'm already way too busy.
Must Comply With All Dietary Guidelines From Qualified Dietitians.

An actual meal is what a meal replacement is. I also need to make sure I'm getting all the vitamins, amino acids, fiber, and other nutrients my body needs when I'm trying to lose weight. It's that easy to find, but I had trouble. Ignore the liquid diet for losing weight. They simply lack intelligence.

All-natural testosterone boosters.
Many of our hormones, particularly testosterone, start to drop as we age as men. In truth, the fitness industry has been looking for safe, natural testosterone supplements for decades as a way to lose weight, but they have not been widely accessible until lately.

In addition to making a guy "a man," testosterone also turns a man into a lean, nasty machine. Increased muscle mass, decreased body fat, higher energy, healthier confidence and sex drive levels, and greater sexual stamina and drive are the key advantages of testosterone.
And as a Prograde Nutrition partner, I wanted to share this all-natural testosterone booster with you.
The Untold Tale of Testosterone and Fat Loss Regulation.

These advantages have made testosterone the fountain of youth for men, and as a result, men all over the world are attempting to increase their testosterone levels.
Nevertheless, using testosterone injections without a prescription is not only prohibited but also has a host of negative side effects, including increased aggression and prostate problems brought on by hormonal imbalances.
Moreover, the testicles, which are the body's primary makers of testosterone, shut down and start to shrink after receiving an injection of exogenous testosterone. To maintain proper hormone levels, your body essentially starts to rely on a weekly shot. This is not a good thing.
The Comprehensive Approach

If you are familiar with holistic health, you will disagree with the aforementioned strategy because there are much better and healthier ways to encourage your body to make testosterone naturally so you won't have to worry about a wide range of adverse effects.

Even though they are enduring the negative effects of low testosterone, many men do not even meet the criteria for legal hormone therapy.

Because of this, it's crucial to look for a natural fat loss remedy if you notice that your testosterone levels are declining as you age and it affects both how you feel and how you appear.

The Scary Truth About Testosterone and Your Metabolism and Why You May Be Getting Fat!

Your body's ability to control how much fat it creates is mostly due to testosterone. Higher body fat levels—which are bad for a man—will be apparent if you have low testosterone levels. Since testosterone is in charge of generating a healthy metabolism, a whole new problem of a lower metabolic rate occurs as men age and as testosterone levels drop.

In layman's terms, low testosterone levels will also hinder your body's capacity to burn calories, which will cause you to accumulate extra fat over days and months.

The news is NOT good.

This implies that millions of men worldwide gain unneeded fat every year, even though natural testosterone supplements may entirely fix the issue and restore the proper body chemistry in these individuals.

One way that men can fight the issue of developing unneeded body fat, which to some appears practically unavoidable, is by naturally increasing their testosterone levels.

Trying to diet didn't work for me.

This is something that men who become motivated, start an exercise regimen, and attempt to eat a good and balanced diet tell me virtually every week. They appear to be moving extremely slowly. If you experience this, you might want to consider taking natural testosterone pills as a solution to your issues with fat loss.

One of the keys to sustained fat loss is increasing your energy expenditure, which you may be able to do with the use of natural testosterone supplements like Prograde's K20. Also, it might help you gain strength, fight minor depression, boost your confidence, and keep a good outlook. The importance of keeping a positive outlook on life when attempting to achieve your goals is often overlooked. Since testosterone is the hormone that creates the specific mindset that men need to achieve their fat goals, nothing else may be able to assist you in doing this.

They appear to be moving extremely slowly. If you experience this, you might want to consider taking natural testosterone pills as a solution to your issues with fat loss.

One of the keys to sustained fat loss is increasing your energy expenditure, which you may be able to do with the use of natural testosterone supplements like Prograde's K20. Also, it might help you gain strength, fight minor depression, boost your confidence, and keep a good outlook. The importance of keeping a positive outlook on life when attempting to achieve your goals is often overlooked. As testosterone is the hormone that develops the specific attitude that men need to attain their fat goals, nothing else may be able to assist you in doing this.

You should keep in mind that there is no need to undersell yourself when there are natural testosterone pills that may assist enhance testosterone levels, allowing you to stop worrying about why you are unable to lose fat.

Your body has to be "reset" if your stamina has diminished, your confidence has dropped, or you simply don't feel like "you" anymore to reclaim the macho "Mojo" necessary for male survival and the secret to loving being a lean, mean, man-machine.

Supplements for Athletes' Nutrition

If you enjoy working out and are interested in discovering the best nutritional supplements for athletes and getting as thin as possible, then you know that there comes a time when you need to stop.

This is especially true for fat loss, which explains the significance of nutritional supplements for athletes.

99.999% of the time, this "wall" is only a dietary shortfall, even though many athletes refer to it as a "wall." This is why it's crucial for every athlete to regularly refill their nutritional stores. Consistent here refers to daily. This is precisely what is necessary to produce the outcomes that each of us seeks.

In actuality, what distinguishes the good from the excellent and the best from the exceptional is access to and knowledge of the best nutritional supplements for athletes. If you want to improve your physical performance while also lowering your body fat percentage, you must concentrate on the dietary components of your exercise program to achieve the best outcomes.

You see, if you don't have access to some of the top-quality nutritional supplements for athletes on the market, you will have to spend more time in the gym, eat more frequently, take more vitamins, and generally spend more time attempting to nourish your body.

I used to be here a few years back. And trust me, it's not a good situation because it only served to waste my time. Instead of trying to chase a calorie to help me lose fat in a post, I could have spent that time doing the things I love to do.

But Everything Has Changed Now.

You do not have to learn the hard way as I did. With the proliferation of supplement retailers both online and offline, it can be challenging to tell which products are best for fat reduction from those that aren't.

In my capacity as an athlete and a partner of Prograde Nutrition, I am aware that I must replenish my body's nutritional needs daily—and not just with food from the grocery store. Instead, I use nutritional supplements designed specifically for athletes, which enable me to consume many more nutrients than I ever could have on my own.

Let's face it, I simply don't want to spend the entire day chewing food at a table to give my body the vitamins and nutrients it needs to keep the leanness that I so dearly value. That would wreck my social life and is just not enjoyable.

Let's now explore some research related to how you will become and maintain a slender body. This is when things start to get dangerous and exciting because you can take action!

The word "gluconeogenesis" is a bad one! Particularly the Following Training

If the term "60-minute window" is unfamiliar to you,
The "60-minute window," for those of you who are unfamiliar, is the period immediately following your workout during which your body is pleading with you to replenish its nutrients, particularly the glycogen that it lost during training.
Glycogen is merely a kind of carbohydrate that is stored but is used up during exercise. When you stop exercising, your body transitions from a fat-burning phase (if you exercised for more than 20 minutes) back into resting mode, when it will need glycogen from your stored energy to function normally.
After your workout, if a sufficient quantity of carbs is not immediately available, your body will initiate a process known as gluconeogenesis.

This is your body's effort to make carbohydrates from sources other than carbohydrates, such as protein.
This implies that as soon as you finish training, your hard-earned muscle may be utilized to replace your glycogen stores!
You don't want this, and it interferes with your efforts to lose weight!
The primary metabolic booster your body possesses, your muscle tissue, is also being consumed as your body starts to digest its muscle tissue to produce carbs. This will hinder your attempts to lose weight and put you on a metabolic cycle analogous to "Robbing Peter to Pay Paul."

Sports nutrition supplements prevent you from running in place!
The best nutritional supplements for athletes can, however, totally solve this issue. This implies that your body will receive the proper protein and carbohydrate types that it needs to recover effectively.

The ability of science to improve our appearance and the amount of fat we can reduce has never been greater than it is now.

CONCLUSION.

READY…SET…GO!

Everyone is aware of what to do now that they have learned how to adjust their lifestyle and lose weight. People read the information and realize they must act and exert effort, but the reality is that people rarely do. You will struggle to start down the path to a healthy life unless you have the self-control to fight the want to eat unhealthy foods and the motivation to eat good foods.

If you don't take that first step, no amount of reading or affirming your ability to succeed will be of any use to you. Both the initial commitment and the ongoing commitment are extremely difficult to maintain.

Most people lose quickly because they are dissatisfied with their outcomes. You will succeed in your mission if you can stay committed, maintain your motivation, and keep setting healthy eating and exercise goals for yourself. You just need to go out there and put in the necessary effort and labor, regardless of your goals—whether they be to reduce weight, build endurance, or improve as an athlete in a particular sport.

Over time, you'll not only mentally get used to your training schedule, but you'll also gain a lot of self-control, discipline, and confidence. You'll also naturally keep a positive outlook, which makes it simple to withstand temptation.

Each person must begin their journey someplace. Instead of striving to go all-out and try to sweat out 10 pounds on the treadmill over a week, setting your goals gradually will be more beneficial. Beginning the process slowly is important, so take a brisk walk to let your body adjust to the more strenuous runs you want to do in the following weeks.

One error beginners make is going all out, which results in injury and prompts them to quickly determine that training is simply too unpleasant and stressful.
Just as before, make a schedule and, if required, speak with a personal trainer about what could be best for you.

There's no need to make the procedure so challenging. If you want to lose weight, all you need is a tiny window of time each day set aside for exercise and to be aware of what you put into your body.
Simply project confidence and work for your objectives. If you are optimistic, you will achieve your goals. Perhaps now is the ideal time to start making that plan and acting so you can start living the super-healthy lifestyle you deserve. As a new season approaches.